Exploring Better Quality of Life:

The Patient's Guide to Bariatric Surgery

MARIA ILIAKOVA, M.D.

Authors: Maria Iliakova, M.D.
Editor: Mira Mdivani

Printed in the United States of America

Library of Congress Cataloging-in-Publication Data

ILIAKOVA, MARIA, 2022
Exploring Better Quality of Life: The Patient's Guide to Bariatric Surgery / Maria Iliakova, M.D.

ISBN: 979-8-9868539-0-1 (Paperback)
ISBN: 979-8-9868539-1-8 (Ebook)

Subjects: Bariatric Surgery | Health – Personal Wellness | Patient advocacy

9 798986 853901

DEDICATIONS

To Mira Mdivani and John Price, M.D.
for essential support and guidance

--Maria Iliakova, M.D

ACKNOWLEDGEMENTS

I would like to thank many dedicated teachers, family members and friends along my path. Mr. Arthur Crumm is an exceptional chemistry teacher who inspired me to pursue science with a questioning mind and sense of humor. Dr. Kathleen Kilway is a force of personality and passion in teaching organic chemistry at UMKC who made a tough subject come alive while also demonstrating female leadership of a university science department. Dr. Chi-Ming Huang and Dr. John Laity both took a chance on me to join their labs, letting me explore interesting ideas with independence. Dr. Lawrence Dreyfus consistently helped to encourage me forward.

At Georgetown, Dr. Mark Danielsen, Dr. Dean Rosenthal, Dr. Simbulan-Rosenthal, Dr. Nathan Edwards, and Dr. Larry Millstein created an innovative learning environment flexible enough to complete a master's degree with a Fulbright research fellowship halfway across the world. Dr. Johannes Jaeger and his pioneering lab at the Center for Genomic Regulation welcomed and supported this Fulbright fellowship and turned the city into a playground.

In medical school at KU, Dean Mark Meyer was a beacon providing relentless support and advice through tough times. Dr. Ivan Damjanov embodied academic medicine with a soul and kindness. Dr. Jennifer Brull demonstrated a robust use of technology in creating a personable medical practice in western Kansas. The phenomenal transplant surgeons of Dr. Timothy Schmitt, Dr. Sean Kumer, and Dr. Atta Nawabi inspired me to go into surgery while on rotation with them. Dr. Randi Ryan, then a surgery resident and now a transplant fellow, gave me her Danskos for a case when I forgot my shoes and the rest is history.

In residency at UMKC and fellowship at Hackensack, there are dozens of people that deserve thanks for countless hours, brain lending, and elbow grease. This includes Dr. John Price who makes damn good surgeons, Dr. Brent Sorensen and Dr. Todd Moore whose technical skills are mastery, Dr. Brook Nelson who is made of sheer will and talent, Dr. Glenn Talboy who gave me a chance to become a surgeon in the first place, Dr. Andrew Benedict who recognizes hard work, Dr. Sean Nix who made sure I survived trauma and ACS rotations, Dr. Barbara Nguyen who always pushes for better, Dr. Megan

McNally who demonstrates how to strive for perfection, Dr. Stanley Augustin who asks the most lasting questions, Dr. Lee Cummings, Dr. Jameson Forster, and Dr. Eddie Island who expect and create miracles, Dr. Dennis Arce who reminded me to slow down and pay attention, Dr. Carol Aylward who makes everyone want to be a plastic surgeon, Dr. Kremer who has a gentle spirit made of steel, Dr. Michael Moncure who never met a stranger and could have made a surgeon out of a rock, Dr. Stanley Sakabu who taught me how to revive a rock, Dr. Dustin Neel who is a compass for navigating ICU and trauma patients, Dr. Karl Stark, Dr. Scott Kujath, and Dr. Jonathan Wilson who made half our residents go into vascular surgery, Dr. Anuj Shah who knows his way around a bad hernia, Dr. Douglas Ewing who made sure I could safely operate even in tough situations, Dr. Sebastian Eid who demonstrates how to keep learning and evolving even as an accomplished surgeon, Dr. Ian Soriano who has already asked more meaningful questions than I'd have considered in a lifetime, Dr. Ben Kulow who always made read and think, and Dr. Douglas Geehan who terrified but ultimately prepared me for boards and open hernias more than he knew, and Julie Porter, NP, who taught me how to take care of bariatric patients. In my family, Lance Gliser, has provided a backbone for multiple moves, years of surgery training, and love along the way, Mira Mdivani, who knows what she's done, Alexey Ayzin who questions everything and cares about purpose above all, Archil Mdivani who shaped all these trajectories, and Colleen Reilly who never lets me get away with anything.

Exploring Better Quality of Life:
The Patient's Guide to Bariatric Surgery

Summary of Contents ─────────────────────────────────

Exploring Better Quality of Life:
The Patient's Guide to Bariatric Surgery

CHAPTER 1: HOW BARIATRIC SURGERY MAY IMPROVE QUALITY OF LIFE

CHAPTER 2: HOW TO PREPARE FOR BARIATRIC SURGERY

CHAPTER 3: THE DAY OF SURGERY

CHAPTER 4: LIFE AFTER BARIATRIC SURGERY

CHAPTER 5: FINAL THOUGHTS FROM A BARIATRIC SURGEON

RESOURCES

CITATIONS

INTRODUCTION: WHAT IS THIS GUIDE and WHO IS IT FOR?

This guide is for you. You may be looking for a way to improve your quality of life. You may be considering surgery for weight management. Maybe you have high blood pressure, diabetes, sleep apnea, or other medical conditions and are considering surgery to help to treat them. This kind of surgery is called bariatric surgery.

In this guide, I will **help to answer questions** you may have, such as:

- How may bariatric surgery improve quality of life?
- Who can benefit from bariatric surgery?
- What bariatric surgeries are done?
- What are the downsides of bariatric surgery?
- How do you prepare for bariatric surgery?
- What happens on the day of surgery?
- What do you do after bariatric surgery?

This guide is not meant to provide medical advice to any specific patient. Because I am a bariatric and general surgeon, I know the importance of having a relationship with a doctor who oversees your specific medical care. This guide is meant to **provide information and support for all patients who are considering or undergoing bariatric surgery.**

TERMS & ABBREVIATIONS

NOTE: These definitions are not universal. They are provided in the context of bariatric surgery practice. This is how I explain these terms to patients when we begin working together.

Bariatric	A term for the field of study including weight, obesity, metabolism, nutrition, physical activity, the interaction of multiple body systems, environment, and public policy.
Bariatric surgery	Surgery done for the purpose of improving quality of life by causing weight loss, metabolic and systematic physical changes.
Body mass index (BMI)	BMI is a ratio of a person's weight to height. A BMI of 40 or more is used as a cutoff to qualify for bariatric surgery. People with a BMI of 35-39 and some health conditions can also quality for bariatric surgery.
Clear liquid diet (CLD)	Clear liquid diet includes liquids that are see-through and easy to swallow. Most clear liquids are drinks, but also includes some jelly products. Examples include water, apply juice, popsicles, and broth.
Duodenal switch surgery (DS)	Also known as a biliopancreatic diversion with duodenal switch, this is a surgery that combines a gastric sleeve surgery plus a long bypass. A new connection is made between the first and last portions of the small intestine to create the long bypass.
Foley catheter	A tube placed into the bladder to allow a person to empty their bladder when they are having trouble doing so on their own.
Full liquid diet (FLD)	Full liquid diet includes all liquids, purees, and puddings that require no chewing. It includes all clear liquids. Examples include baby food and yogurt.
Gastric sleeve surgery	In this surgery, also called a sleeve, approximately 70-

80% of the stomach is removed. The remaining stomach is a skinny tube that looks like a sleeve, hence the name.

Gastric band surgery

During gastric band surgery, a band made of silicone or plastic is placed around the top of the stomach. It connects to tubing and a port that is placed just underneath the skin on the abdomen. This port can be used to add or remove water from the tubing to make the band tighter or looser around the stomach.

Gastric bypass surgery

Also known as a Roux-en-Y gastric bypass, during this surgery, part of the stomach is disconnected from the rest and reconnected to the small intestine. This creates a new route for food that bypasses part of the stomach and small intestine, hence the name bypass.

NSAID

Also known as non-steroidal anti-inflammatory drugs, NSAIDs are a class of medications that include Ibuprofen, Aleve, Advil, Motrin, and Aspirin. These medications wear away the lining of the stomach and intestines. Using these medications increases the risk of ulcers, especially with a bypass surgery.

Pre-authorization

Also known as prior authorization, this is the process that health insurance companies require to approve a bariatric surgery ahead of time.

Post-operative

Also known as post-op, this is the time period after surgery.

Soft diet

This diet, also called mushy or mechanical soft, includes food that is soft or mushy enough that it can be eaten without much chewing. The soft diet includes most mashed and ground foods, as well as all foods on the clear and full liquid diets.

Nutrient

A general term that includes vitamins, micronutrients, and electrolytes. Examples include Vitamin D, B-complex vitamins, calcium, iron, and potassium.

Chapter 1

How Bariatric Surgery May Improve Quality of Life

I.   Bariatric Care is General Health Care

First things first: Is bariatrics all about weight loss?

No. Bariatric care is general health care. While weight and metabolism are at the core of bariatrics, this field is a crossroads of genetics, nutrition, metabolism, the interaction of many body systems, environment, and public policy.

Bariatric care is both medical and surgical. Many kinds of doctors provide bariatric care, such as primary care doctors, bariatric surgeons, endocrinologists, and orthopedic surgeons. There are also many related professionals involved in bariatric health care such as nutritionists, mental health specialists, physical therapists, coordinators, fitness experts, advocates and patients themselves. Most bariatric care extends beyond the walls of a hospital or clinic to involve support from your family and friends.

The purpose of bariatric care is to provide people with a way to improve their health and quality of life.

II. Bariatric Surgery Can Change the Medications You Take, How You Feel, Your Medical Conditions, and Your Weight

The purpose of bariatric health care is to improve a person's quality of life.

Bariatric surgery is done to allow people to do things like:

- Decrease the number of blood pressure medications taken
- Walk up and down the stairs more easily if you have arthritis
- Dance at a wedding without hurting
- Walk, bike, or swim with greater ease when you feel like it
- Bend without having to hold your breath
- Decrease reflux symptoms
- Sleep at night without snoring
- Decrease the number of diabetes medications taken
- Lose weight
- Feel better about overall physical and mental health

Bariatric surgery causes weight loss by changing how much a person can eat, how food is absorbed and digested, metabolism, and how different body systems interact with each other. As a result, people often experience positive changes in the management of their blood pressure, diabetes, arthritis, reflux, sleep apnea, cholesterol, heart disease, and mental health. While bariatric surgery is not right for every patient, it is effective for some people who want to lose weight and to treat some medical conditions.

In the next section, we will discuss what to expect from bariatric surgery.

III.   Bariatric Surgery Is Not for Everyone

Even though bariatric surgery is very useful, it is important to recognize that bariatric surgery is not a magic bullet. Even after bariatric surgery, it is important to pay attention to nutrition, stay active, and to keep track of your overall health for the rest of your life. We will discuss the details of who qualifies for surgery and BMI in Chapter 2.

Bariatric surgery also has some limitations. It is **not** realistic to expect the following from bariatric surgery:

- Losing weight below a BMI of 25,
- A guarantee to reach or maintain a specific goal weight,
- Avoiding damage to your body done by a specific health condition, smoking, or drug use,
- A promise that a specific health condition will improve or be cured, OR
- A guarantee that you will not experience a complication after surgery.

While bariatric surgery is an appropriate option for many people looking to lose weight and treat some medical conditions, it is not a good option for everyone. Bariatric surgery may not be a good choice for people with:

- BMI over 40 who are healthy and not seeking to lose weight
- BMI under 35, except in specific cases
- Medical conditions that would make surgery unsafe, such as end-stage lung disease, severe heart failure, and portal hypertension
- Current pregnancy
- Dependency on drugs or alcohol

- Some mental health conditions
- Low social support

In some of these cases, bariatric surgery may become an option at another time if these conditions change.

In the next section, we will discuss what to expect from bariatric surgery.

IV.   What to Expect from Bariatric Surgery

The goal of bariatric surgery is to improve quality of life. These improvements may be physical and mental. It is reasonable to expect that bariatric surgery may help you to:

- Decrease the number of blood pressure medications you take
- Walk up and down the stairs more easily if you have arthritis
- Decrease reflux symptoms
- Sleep at night without snoring
- Decrease the number of diabetes medications you take
- Lose weight
- Stop your heart disease from getting worse
- Feel better about your overall health
- Repair fatty liver disease not caused by alcohol

If any of these expectations relate to you, bariatric surgery may be a good fit for you.

Bariatric surgery requires some changes to your life. It is important to be ready for these changes before choosing to have surgery. These are changes such as:

- Regular follow up with your bariatric surgery team and primary care doctor,
- Keeping track of your nutrition with increased water intake, daily supplements, smaller meals more often throughout the day and keeping a healthy diet,
- Avoiding smoking for life, especially with gastric bypass or duodenal switch surgery,
- Avoid Ibuprofen and this entire class of medications called NSAIDS if you have had a gastric bypass or duodenal switch surgery,

- Staying physically active for life, AND

- Getting regular physical and mental health care.

When considering bariatric surgery, it is important to know what to expect from surgery. As you can see, you play the most important role in deciding what you want out of bariatric surgery. You also have the most important role in your life after surgery. If you and your surgeon decide that bariatric surgery fits your needs and expectations, you can expect support along the way to reaching a better quality of life.

In the next section, we will discuss the process of preparing for bariatric surgery.

Chapter 2

How to Prepare for Bariatric Surgery

I. How to Decide When Bariatric Surgery May Be Right for You

You may consider bariatric surgery if you want to improve your quality of life. Bariatric surgery may help you achieve any of these things:

- Lower the number of blood pressure medications you take
- Walk up and down the stairs more easily if you have arthritis
- Decrease reflux symptoms
- Sleep at night without snoring
- Decrease the number of diabetes medications you take
- Lose weight
- Stop your heart disease from getting worse
- Bend without having to hold your breath
- Feel better about your overall health

BMI, body mass index, is used as a cutoff to qualify for bariatric surgery. BMI is a measure calculated using a person's height and weight. The BMI is not a perfect measure. However, at this time it is the standard used in the U.S. to decide which individuals to approve for bariatric surgery.

In general, there are two (2) ways to be approved for bariatric surgery:

1. Have a BMI of 40 or over, OR
2. Have a BMI of 35-39 and at least one of several specific health conditions, listed further in this section.

To get an idea whether you may qualify for bariatric surgery, you may start by measuring your BMI. If you know your height and weight, you can use an online BMI calculator from the NIH, National Institutes of Health at this link: https://www.nhlbi.nih.gov/health/educational/lose_wt/BMI/bmicalc.htm. You can also ask your doctor's office to calculate your BMI.

A person who is 5 foot 4 inches tall has a BMI of 40 at a weight of 232 pounds.
A person who is 6 feet tall has a BMI of 40 at a weight of 294 pounds.
There is no difference in BMI for men or women, age, fitness level, or overall health.

If you have a BMI between 35 and 39, you can still qualify for approval for bariatric surgery if you have any of the following medical conditions:

- Diabetes
- High blood pressure
- Sleep apnea, asthma, and related chronic breathing problems
- Fatty liver disease that is not caused by alcohol
- Arthritis
- High cholesterol
- Heart disease
- Chronic depression
- Some types of urinary incontinence

This is a current list of conditions covered by most health insurance plans at this time and may change in the future.

A person who is 5 foot 4 inches tall has a BMI of 35 at a weight of 204 pounds.

A person who is 6 feet tall has a BMI of 35 at a weight of 258 pounds.

To recap, the two main ways to quality for approval of bariatric surgery are to:

1. Have a BMI of 40 or over, OR

2. Have a BMI of 35-39 and at least one of the following health conditions: Diabetes, high blood pressure, sleep apnea, asthma, chronic breathing problems, fatty liver not caused by alcohol, arthritis, high cholesterol, heart disease, chronic depression, and stress urinary incontinence

If you meet these either of these conditions, you can ask your health insurance company to cover the cost of your bariatric surgery. If you do not meet these conditions, you may still qualify for bariatric surgery, but you may have to pay out of pocket.

Every insurance company has different rules to qualify for bariatric surgery. These rules vary by plan and state. To find out your specific qualifying BMI, medical conditions, and other information about costs and coverage, check with your insurance company directly. If you are already working with a bariatric surgery team, it is a good idea to ask to help you navigate cost and insurance coverage.

Bariatric surgery may not be a good choice for people with:

- BMI over 40 and are healthy and not seeking to lose weight
- BMI under 35, except in specific cases
- Medical conditions that would make surgery unsafe, such as end-stage lung disease, severe heart failure, and portal hypertension

- Current pregnancy

- Dependency on drugs or alcohol

- Some mental health conditions

- Low social support

Even in some of these cases above, bariatric surgery may become a good option in the future. Ultimately, the decision to offer and choose surgery is a conversation between a patient and their bariatric surgery team.

Though BMI is used as a cutoff for bariatric surgery coverage, I think the most important question to ask yourself is about quality of life and your own expectations. Ask yourself: What do I want out of it?

Bariatric surgery cannot guarantee a specific result. It is a good option for people wanting to lose and maintain a lower weight. It is also a good option for treating many health conditions such as high blood pressure, diabetes, non-alcoholic fatty liver disease, and high cholesterol. Bariatric surgery is also useful for treating sleep apnea, arthritis, heart disease, reflux, and chronic depression. Treatment of these conditions can mean fewer medications, easier movement, and better mental health.

If you would like to find out if you qualify for bariatric surgery or find a program in your area, start by talking with your primary care doctor. There are many resources online to help you find a bariatric surgeon in your area. Many bariatric surgery programs offer online and in-person seminars for people to learn about what they offer and how to get started.

Next, we will review the different kinds of bariatric surgeries done in the U.S.

II.   The Different Kinds of Bariatric Surgeries

There is no one kind of bariatric surgery that is the best. No surgery is perfect for everybody. Each patient's goals and health matter most in deciding which surgery is the best for him or her. The decision to offer and choose a bariatric surgery is a discussion patient and their bariatric surgeon.

Before we discuss the specific types of bariatric surgeries, recognize that surgery is not a magic bullet. Bariatric surgery changes your physical body, metabolism, and how different body systems interact with each other. Whether your quality of life improves or not depends as much on surgery as on your nutrition, activity, and overall mental and physical health after surgery.

We break down surgeries into two main categories: restrictive and metabolic. Restrictive surgeries change the size and shape of the stomach. This makes the stomach smaller and feel fuller faster. Metabolic surgeries change how the body absorbs and metabolizes food and how different body systems work together. In practice, all bariatric surgeries are both restrictive and metabolic. Specific bariatric surgeries are more one than the other.

The most common bariatric surgeries performed in the US include the following:

- Gastric sleeve (also known as sleeve)
- Gastric bypass (also known as Roux-en-Y gastric bypass)
- Duodenal switch (also known as Biliopancreatic Diversion with Duodenal Switch)
- Gastric band
- Revision surgery

Gastric Sleeve Surgery

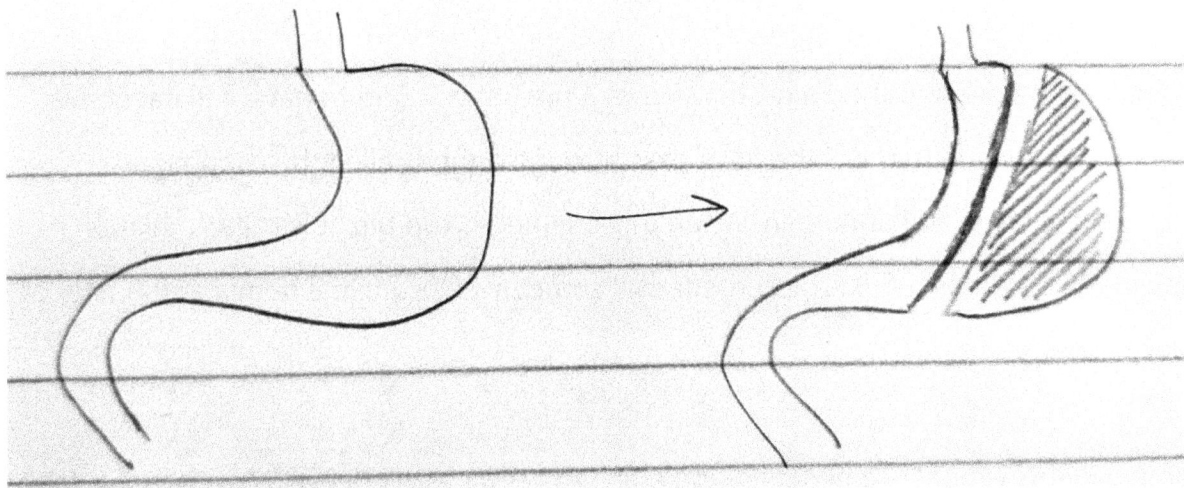

During gastric sleeve surgery, approximately 70-80% of the stomach is removed. The remaining stomach is a skinny tube that looks like a sleeve. That is why this surgery is called a sleeve.

The gastric sleeve is a restrictive surgery, meaning that there is less space for food to go. As a result, the stomach feels full faster. The sleeve also changes how the body signals hunger and fullness. It not only affects these hormones but also changes how the body metabolizes food.

A patient can expect to lose about 40-60% of overweight body weight with a gastric sleeve. If 100 pounds overweight, he or she can expect to lose 40-60 pounds.

After a gastric sleeve, most patients find it uncomfortable to eat or drink very much at once. Eating smaller, more frequent meals and drinking often throughout the day is important after surgery. These changes are meant to last for a lifetime. In the year after surgery, most bariatric surgery teams follow up with their sleeve patients once every few months, and then once a year after that.

Sometimes before or during a gastric sleeve, a patient is found to have a hiatal hernia. There is an opening that lets the food pass through a tube called the esophagus between the chest and abdomen. When this opening is too big, it is called a hiatal hernia, which causes reflux. The surgeon will sometimes fix a hiatal hernia at the time of sleeve surgery.

Some patients experience negative side effects after a gastric sleeve. Most patients feel some nausea or bloating immediately after surgery, but this typically goes away in several days. Some patients have reflux that is new or becomes worse after sleeve surgery. Some patients regain weight over time. There may be other problems, depending on your specific surgery and overall health. It is important to have regular follow-up with your primary care doctor and your bariatric surgery team, especially if experiencing any of these problems after gastric sleeve surgery.

Gastric Bypass Surgery (also known as Roux-en-Y Gastric Bypass)

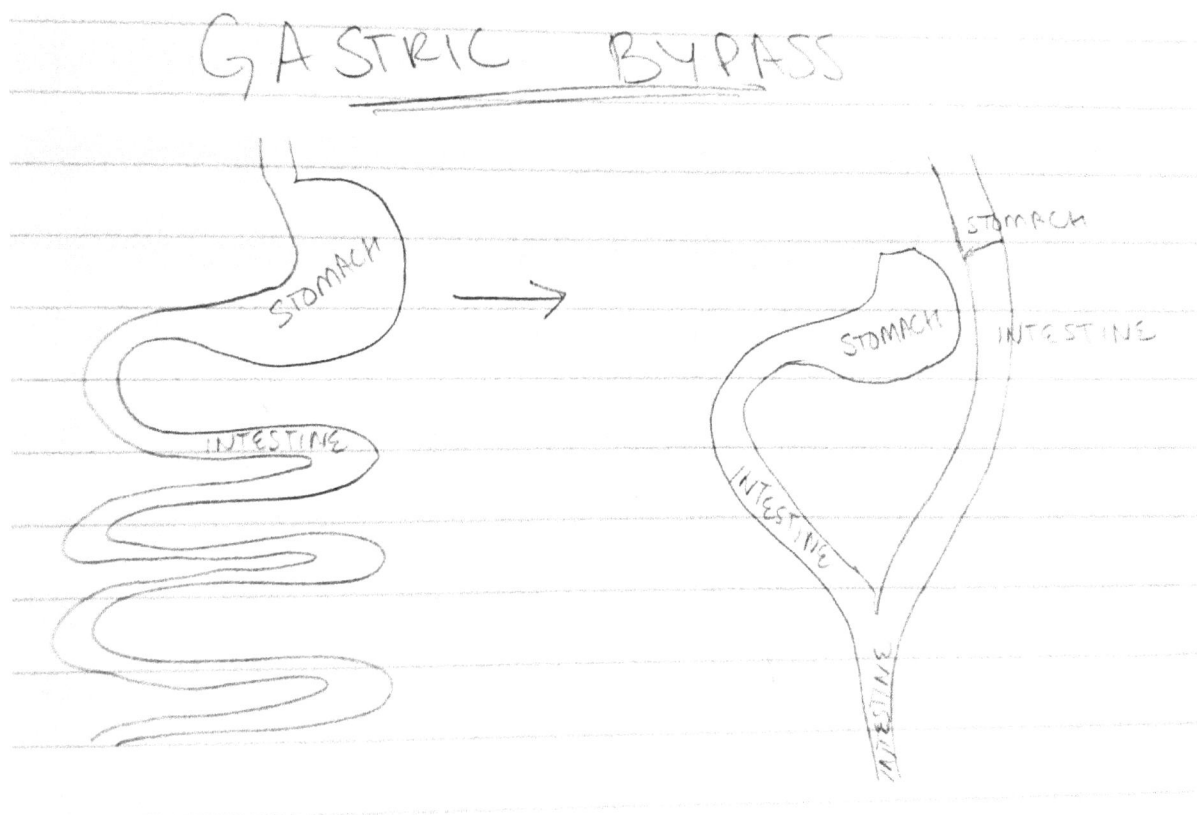

During gastric bypass surgery, part of the stomach is disconnected from the rest and reconnected to the small intestine. This creates a new route for food that bypasses part of the stomach and intestine. The gastric bypass is a restrictive and metabolic surgery.

There is less space for food to go in the stomach. As a result, it feels full faster. The bypass also changes how the body absorbs and processes food, even more so than the gastric sleeve surgery. It also has a bigger impact on changing how body systems work together. The bypass may be helpful in treating diabetes, high blood pressure, reflux, high cholesterol, and heart disease.

A patient can expect to lose about 60-80% of overweight body weight with a gastric bypass. If 100 pounds overweight, a patient can expect to lose 60-80 pounds.

After a gastric bypass, most patients find it uncomfortable to eat or drink very much at once. Eating smaller, more frequent meals and drinking often throughout the day is important after surgery. These changes are intended to last a lifetime. In the year after surgery, most bariatric surgery teams follow up with their gastric bypass patients once every few months, and then once a year after that.

Some patients experience negative side effects after a gastric bypass. Some patients feel nausea or bloating immediately after surgery, but this typically goes away in several days. Bypass surgery causes less nutrient absorption. It is easy to be low on some vitamins and micronutrients if supplements are not taken every day and tracked with regular visits to the doctor.

After a bypass surgery, there is also higher risk of an intestinal blockage that may require a surgery to fix. Smoking and using medications like Ibuprofen after a bypass surgery wear away the lining of the new connection between the stomach and intestine. This can cause an ulcer that can be painful and make a patient very sick. Some patients regain weight in the long term, but this is less common than with a gastric sleeve. There may be other problems, depending on your specific surgery and overall health. It is important to have regular follow-up with a primary care doctor and bariatric surgery team, especially if experiencing any of these problems after gastric bypass surgery.

Duodenal Switch (also known as Biliopancreatic Diversion with Duodenal Switch)

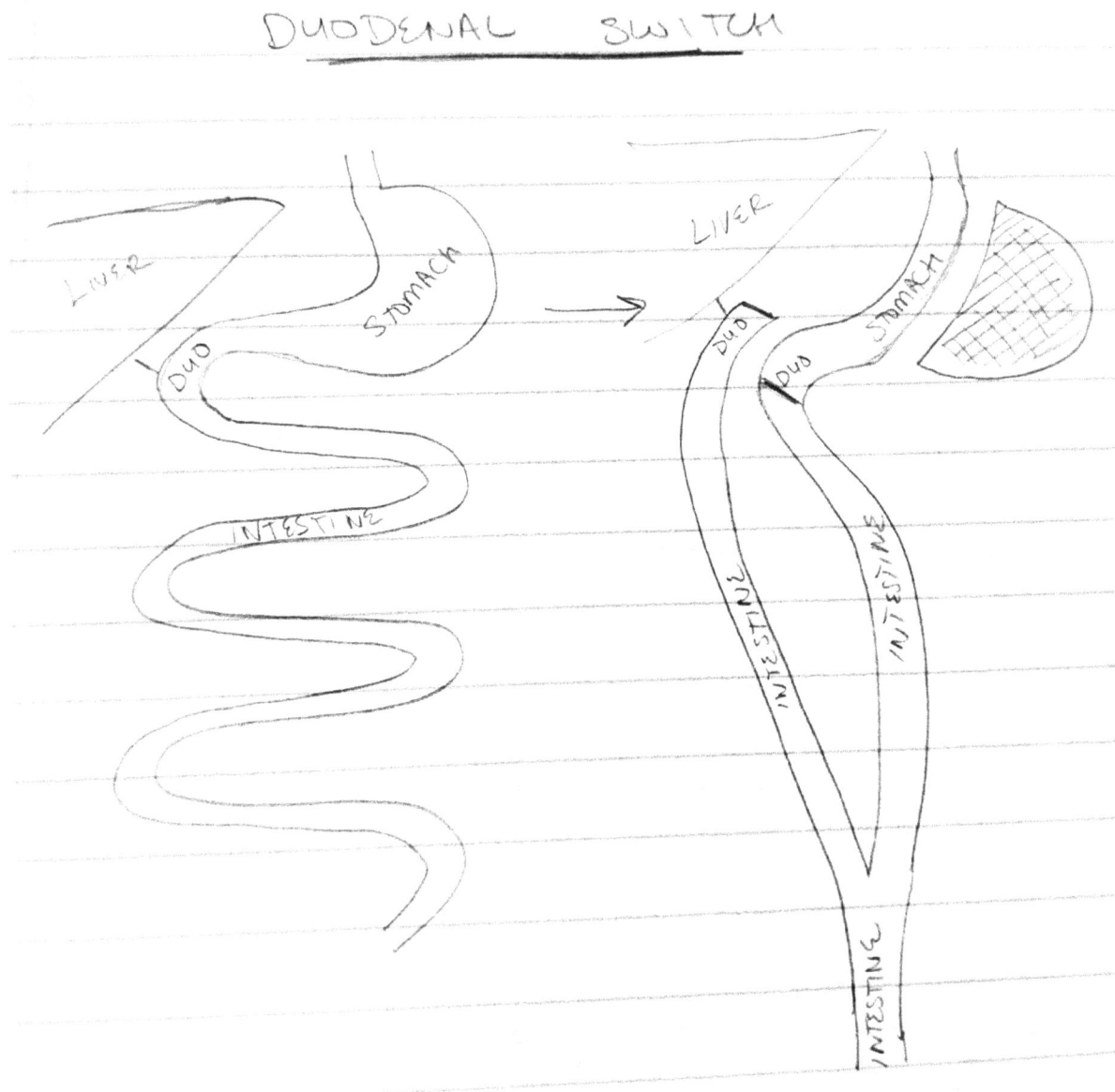

During duodenal switch surgery, approximately 70-80% of the stomach is removed and a new connection is made between the small intestines that skips most of it. This surgery is a combination of a sleeve plus a long bypass. The duodenal switch is both a restrictive and metabolic surgery.

There is less space for food to go in your stomach. As a result, it feels full faster. The bypass also changes how the body absorbs and processes food, even more so than the gastric bypass. It also has a bigger impact on changing how body systems work together. The duodenal switch may be helpful in treating diabetes, high blood pressure, reflux, high cholesterol, and heart disease.

A patient can expect to lose over 80% of overweight body weight with a duodenal switch surgery. If 100 pounds overweight, a patient can expect to lose over 80 pounds.

After a duodenal switch, most patients find it uncomfortable to eat or drink very much at once. Eating smaller, more frequent meals and drinking often throughout the day is important after surgery. These changes are intended to last for a lifetime. In the year after surgery, most bariatric surgery teams follow up with their duodenal switch patients once every few months, and then once a year after that.

Some patients experience negative side effects after a duodenal switch. Some patients feel nausea or bloating immediately after surgery, but this typically goes away in several days. Bypass surgery causes less food and nutrient absorption. It is easy to be low on some vitamins and micronutrients if supplements are not taken every day and tracked with regular visits to the doctor. Some patients have diarrhea after surgery, most of which can be treated with medications or changing foods.

After a duodenal switch surgery, there is higher risk of an intestinal blockage that may require a surgery to fix. Some patients lose too much weight or have diarrhea, which can sometimes be treated with medications and lifestyle changes. In some cases, another surgery is needed. Some patients regain weight in the long term, but this is rare. There may be other problems, depending on your specific surgery and overall health. It is important to have regular follow-up with a primary care doctor and bariatric surgery team, especially if experiencing any of these problems after duodenal switch surgery.

Gastric Band Surgery

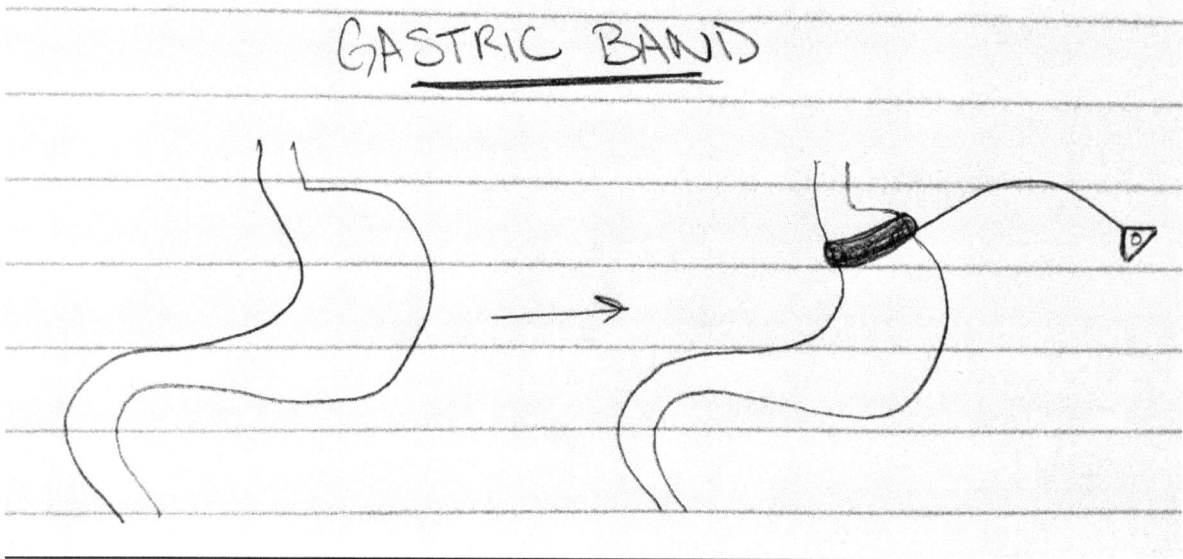

GASTRIC BAND

During gastric band surgery, a band made of silicone or plastic is placed around part of the top of the stomach. It connects to tubing and a port that is placed just underneath the skin on the abdomen. This port allows a health care provider to add or remove water from the tubing connected to pockets around the band. This causes the band to become tighter or looser around the stomach.

The gastric band is a restrictive surgery because there is less space for food to go in your stomach. As a result, it feels full faster.

Weight loss with a gastric band is not consistent. Some patients lose up to 40% of their overweight body weight. If 100 pounds overweight, a patient can lose up to 40 pounds.

After a gastric band, most patients find it uncomfortable to eat or drink very much at once. Eating smaller, more frequent meals and drinking often throughout the day is important after surgery. Fluid in the band can be added or removed to make the band tighter or looser over the time. In the year after surgery, most surgeons follow up with their band patients once every few months, and then at least once a year after that.

Some patients experience negative side effects to a gastric band. Some patients feel nausea or bloating after surgery. Gastric bands often need to be managed by adding or removing fluid from the band over time. Bands can also move and cause problems requiring the band be adjusted or removed.

After gastric band surgery, many patients do not lose significant weight or regain weight over time. As a result, bands are best used in limited circumstances. There may be other problems, depending on your specific surgery and overall health. It is important to have regular follow-up with a primary care doctor and bariatric surgery team, especially if you experience any of these problems after gastric band surgery.

Revision Bariatric Surgery

Bariatric surgeries are meant to be done once in a lifetime. However, this not always possible. Some patients have problems after surgery like regaining weight or worsening reflux. Some of these conditions can be managed with medications or lifestyle changes. Some require surgery. When another surgery is done, it is called a revision surgery and is unique to each patient. These surgeries require careful consideration between the patient and their bariatric surgery team.

Some Other Things to Consider About Bariatric Surgery and Following Weight Loss

We have discussed gastric sleeves, gastric bypasses, duodenal switches, gastric bands, and revisional bariatric surgeries. As you can see, there is no one perfect surgery and no one surgery that fits the needs of every patient. The decision to have a specific bariatric surgery depends on you and your bariatric surgeon.

After surgery, most surgeons ask their patients to stay on a liquid diet for a specific amount of time. The exact liquid diet and length of time to stay on it varies by surgeon and by surgery. We will discuss diets after bariatric surgery in more detail in Chapter 4.

Patients who lose weight after bariatric surgery sometimes have loose skin because of weight loss. In some cases, patients may consider plastic surgery to remove or contour loose skin. This is entirely up to the patient. If you have questions about body shape after bariatric surgery, discuss this with your bariatric surgery team.

In the next section, we will walk through step-by-step the process to prepare for bariatric surgery.

III.   Preparing for Surgery

Now that you may be considering bariatric surgery, we will review the steps to getting from square one to surgery. This is an overview of the steps required to get health insurance approval for bariatric surgery. This process is not specific to any one health insurance plan. For specific plan details, contact your health insurance company directly.

The process to get approved for bariatric surgery usually take between 3 to 8 months. These are the general steps you need to take to get approved for your bariatric surgery:

- See your primary care doctor for an evaluation
- Go to a patient education event with a bariatric surgery team
- Schedule an appointment with a bariatric surgery team
- Discuss your goals and options with a bariatric surgeon
- Write down the ways that you have tried to lose weight in the past
- Meet with a nutritionist
- See a mental health specialist for an evaluation
- Get an EKG, an electrical study of your heart
- Get lab work done
- See a specialist for an evaluation, if needed
- File paperwork with your health insurance company for approval for your surgery

See your primary care doctor for an evaluation

First, go see your primary care doctor. Your doctor will evaluate your overall health. Discuss your goals with them and why you are considering bariatric surgery. If your doctor think you could be a good fit, they will refer you to a bariatric surgery team.

Sometimes you will see a bariatric surgeon first and go see a primary care doctor second. That is fine. The order is not important.

In your discussion, you may find that bariatric surgery is not the right choice for you. You can still discuss medications and lifestyle changes that may work for you. Ask about these options even if bariatric surgery is not on the table.

Go to a patient education event with a bariatric surgery team

Many bariatric surgery teams host education events and seminars online or in person. These seminars help people learn about bariatric surgery. The surgery team will introduce themselves and explain the process of bariatric surgery. You will also learn how to schedule an appointment with the bariatric surgery team, which is the next step.

Schedule an appointment with a bariatric surgery team

When you schedule an appointment with a bariatric surgery team, you will meet with several people, including the bariatric surgeon, nurses, coordinators, nutritionists and mental health specialists. In most cases, you will work closely with a coordinator, who will help you to set a timeline, schedule appointments, and complete paperwork to help you get approved for bariatric surgery.

You may discuss the cost of your care with your bariatric surgery team. You may qualify for some or all care to be covered by your health insurance company, but this will vary by policy, surgery, and your specific situation.

As part of this process, you may decide that surgery is not the right choice for you or to try medications or lifestyle changes first. That is a valid choice at any time along your path. The bariatric surgery team may be able to provide this care or can refer you to someone who can.

Discuss your goals and options with a bariatric surgeon

When you meet with the bariatric surgeon, you will discuss your overall health, goals, and your expectations. The surgeon will explain which surgeries are appropriate, if any fit your needs. Keep in mind that not all surgeries are a good option for every person. Also be aware that bariatric surgery is not right for everyone.

Your surgeon should be able to discuss treatment options besides surgery, such as not having surgery. He or she should also be able to review the risks of surgery with you. If the surgeon offers you a bariatric surgery, the choice to have surgery is yours alone.

You will likely have another visit with your bariatric surgeon once your surgery date is closer. At this pre-surgery visit, ask about which medications you should take and not take on the day of surgery. You should also ask about any restrictions on eating or drinking before your surgery. Make sure that you understand your instructions for the day of surgery so that you can follow them and stay safe on the day of surgery.

Write down ways that you have tried to lose weight in the past

You will be asked to write down or discuss how you have tried to lose weight in the past. This includes any programs, medications, diets, or other methods you have tried. It is important to be as specific and complete as possible.

This question is a standard in the approval process asked by health insurance companies to find out if you qualify for bariatric surgery. This can be a difficult or uncomfortable question to answer. Ask your bariatric surgery team to help you with this step.

Most of the time, patients are asked to avoid gaining weight before surgery. There are many ways bariatric surgery teams can support patients in this, so do not be afraid to ask for help. Some programs will ask you to participate in a weight management program, even if you have done so in the past. This is also required by some health insurance plans to be approved for bariatric surgery.

Meet with a nutritionist and prepare for changes with bariatric surgery

Meeting with a nutritionist is a great way to learn about your nutrition and expectations of what to eat before and after bariatric surgery. You will talk about how and what you eat, your water and nutrient intake, and any diets you have tried. You will also be able to plan your nutrition for the future. Most importantly, you will learn about how your eating will change after surgery.

Most bariatric surgery teams ask patients to stay on a liquid diet after surgery. Some ask for this before surgery as well. Liquid diets vary by specific type and length of time. Ask your nutritionist about the diet plan that you will be asked to follow before and after your surgery. Make sure that you understand the different types of liquid diets, what you can eat while you are on them, and how long you will be on them.

We will review the types of liquid diets in Chapter 4.

You may meet with the nutritionist once or multiple times. Most health insurance plans require patients to meet with a nutritionist a specific number of times before getting approved for bariatric surgery. Ask about this number to make sure that you reach it.

See a mental health specialist for an evaluation

Going through bariatric surgery and taking care of yourself afterwards can be tough, both physically and mentally. It is a team effort with every patient to make sure we are set up for success.

A visit with a qualified mental health specialist is an important part of getting ready for the changes following bariatric surgery. This visit helps you to discuss your goals, concerns, and to find out if you have enough support in your life to go through bariatric surgery safely and accomplish your goals in the longer term. During this visit, it is important to identify any reasons to avoid or delay bariatric surgery, when needed. A visit with a mental health specialist is required by most health insurance plans to be approved for bariatric surgery.

Having a mental health condition does not stop you from qualifying for bariatric surgery. In fact, many people with mental health conditions go through surgery safely and improve the quality of their lives. It is important to make sure your mental health is discussed and properly supported before and after bariatric surgery.

Get an EKG, an electrical study of your heart

In most cases before bariatric surgery, you will be asked to get a study of your heart called an EKG, also known as an electrocardiogram. During the EKG, small pads will be placed along your body to measure the electrical activity of your heart. You do not feel the study when it is done.

This study helps to find any heart problems you may have. It is not a complete picture of your heart function. If there is a problem seen on your EKG, you may need to have more tests done or to see a heart specialist, called a cardiologist.

Get lab work done

In most cases before bariatric surgery, you will be asked to get some lab work done. This involves taking a blood sample to be able to test it for things like your hemoglobin, creatinine, electrolytes, HbA1c, and vitamin levels. This helps to find out if there are any problems that need to be taken care of before surgery. These labs also help to set a baseline that can be used to compare against in the future.

The labs drawn vary by your medical history and by health insurance plan. For specific labs that apply to you, discuss this with your bariatric surgery team.

See a specialist for an evaluation, if needed

In some cases, it is very important to see a specialist doctor in addition to your bariatric surgery team before bariatric surgery. You may need to see a specialist if you have high blood pressure, diabetes, sleep apnea or other medical conditions. You may already know about one of these conditions or one may be found during the evaluations you are undergoing before bariatric surgery

If you have diabetes, you may be asked to see an endocrinologist. If you have a heart condition, you may be asked to see a cardiologist. If you snore at night or have trouble sleeping, you may be asked to complete a sleep study.

During these visits with your specialist doctor, you will discuss medications or other treatments. Take time to ask how these medications or treatments may change after surgery. You and your specialist doctor will work together to help make you as safe and healthy as possible to undergo bariatric surgery.

File paperwork with your health insurance company for approval for surgery

As you can see, there are a lot of "t"s to cross and "i"s to dot to get approved for bariatric surgery from a health insurance company. Along the way, you and your bariatric surgery team work together to make sure that you are supported and prepared for surgery.

Health insurance companies ask for this paperwork to make sure that you qualify for surgery based on their rules. This is called "pre-authorization" or "prior authorization". Your coordinator from the bariatric surgery team will help you to stay on schedule to complete all the steps and to get your paperwork filed. Work with your coordinator to set a timeline and get all the support you need to get these steps done.

Along this path, you may decide not to have surgery. There are still medication and lifestyle options to explore. Discuss these with your bariatric surgery team. They may be able to provide some of this care or refer you to a doctor or team who does.

Your bariatric pre-surgery checklist

There are many steps before bariatric surgery to make sure it is the right choice for you. You and your bariatric surgery team will work together to set you up for success.

Here is the overview checklist of things to do before your bariatric surgery:

- See your primary care doctor for an evaluation
- Go to a patient education event with a bariatric surgery team
- Schedule an appointment with a bariatric surgery team
- Discuss your goals and options with a bariatric surgeon
- Write down the ways that you have tried to lose weight in the past
- Meet with a nutritionist and prepare for your nutrition changes after surgery
- See a mental health specialist for an evaluation
- Get an EKG, an electrical study of your heart
- Get lab work done
- See a specialist for an evaluation, if needed
- File paperwork with your health insurance company for approval for your surgery

Along this path, keep your goals in mind, ask questions, and prepare yourself. Use these people and resources to know ahead of time what to expect from your surgery, your nutrition changes, and how to stay safe and healthy before and after surgery.

Once your insurance provider approves surgery, your next step will be set a date for your surgery with your surgeon and prepare for this day.

What to know before your day of bariatric surgery

In general, you will want to know the following before the day of surgery:

- Where and when to go for surgery
- Which medications to take and which not to take on the day of surgery
- When to stop eating and drinking before surgery
- How long you are expected to stay in the hospital after surgery
- Who your support system will be at home

The amount of time you spend in the hospital after bariatric surgery depends on your surgery, your overall health, and how you recover. In some cases, patients can go home the day of surgery. In many cases, patients stay overnight or longer after bariatric surgery. If you have trouble drinking, controlling pain, urinating, nausea or any other problems after surgery, your stay may be longer.

Do not forget that at any time before surgery, you can decide not to have surgery. If this is the case, discuss this with your bariatric surgery team.

In the next section, we will discuss building a support system for yourself with allies before bariatric surgery.

The changes you can expect with bariatric surgery will be both mentally and physical. It takes a village to support a person through these changes.

Before undergoing bariatric surgery, it is important to identify people that will support you throughout this process. Even with a supportive bariatric surgery team on your side, there are many important allies to help along the way, including:

- Primary care doctors
- Specialist doctors
- Nutritionists
- Mental health specialists
- Family
- Friends
- Other bariatric surgery patients

Primary care doctors

Primary care doctors often have long-standing relationships with their patients. These doctors are true quarterbacks for their patients.

Your primary care doctor can provide with a referral to a bariatric surgery team and guidance throughout the process. Your relationship with this doctor is important because they will continue to manage your overall health long-term. Your primary care doctor is an excellent resource for your health care before and after bariatric surgery.

Specialist doctors

Specialist doctors provide care for many bariatric patients. Their expertise is important in treating patients with complex medical conditions. Specialist doctors often play a crucial role in helping patients to consider whether bariatric surgery is a good option for them. These doctors belong to a strong support network for bariatric patients before and after surgery.

Nutritionists

Often the unsung heroes of bariatrics, a nutritionist can help a patient figure out their diet before and after bariatric surgery, supplements to take after surgery, and how to stay on track with nutrition for life. This person can help you prepare for the changes ahead. Work with your nutritionist to know what to eat and drink, how much, and how to keep track of your nutrition before and after bariatric surgery.

Your nutritionist can also be a life-long resource for maintaining your nutrition after bariatric surgery. This person can help you fix the nutrition problems you may face. Your nutritionist is one of your biggest supporters along the bariatric care path.

Mental health specialists

Unfortunately, there is still stigma surrounding bariatrics and obesity. People at all sizes should be treated with dignity and respect. Weight, BMI, and most health conditions are determined by a combination of genetics, nutrition, activity, environment, and policy that no one individual can fully control. People considering bariatric surgery often experience stigma and life conditions that may cause stress, anxiety or depression. It is important to identify these mental health conditions and to start addressing them before surgery.

Meeting with a mental health specialist is a chance to identify things that need to be addressed and the resources in your life. Some people worry about qualifying for bariatric surgery with a mental health condition. Patient with mental health conditions undergo bariatric surgery and may experience better quality of life. It is important to find support for mental health throughout the process and for the rest of your life. Meeting with a mental health specialist regularly can be an important source of support before and after bariatric surgery. Work remains to be done to improve access to mental health support.

Family

It is difficult to go through bariatric surgery and recovery alone. Having a family member that can support you through surgery and life afterwards can be helpful to reaching your goals and improving your quality of life after surgery. Sometimes you will find family members who would like to go on this journey with you or who have had bariatric surgery themselves. Family members can support by listening to you, witnessing your experiences, and taking actions to help you if needed.

Even with family support, you may consider friends and other patients that have gone through bariatric surgery as part of your support system.

Friends

Friends can be a unique source of support for a person undergoing bariatric surgery and through the changes that follow. You may be surprised that some of your friends have had or considered bariatric surgery. While sharing any information about your health is always a personal decision, it is important to identify friends that can help support you throughout this process. Friends may support you by sharing your celebrations and struggles, witnessing your experiences, and taking actions to help you if needed.

Other bariatric surgery patients

Currently, approximately a quarter of a million people undergo bariatric surgery in the U.S every year. Many of these people belong to support groups in their bariatric surgery programs, or other group online or in person. These groups are a treasure trove of experiences, resources, and support for each other and anyone considering bariatric surgery.

Consider looking for support from patient groups early on to help guide your expectations of bariatric surgery. You may ask your bariatric surgery team if there are any patient groups you can join before or after surgery. Patient groups are a strong support system even for those with active family and friend support.

In the next chapter, we will discuss what it is like to have surgery.

Chapter 3

The Day of Surgery

I.   What to Expect the Day of Bariatric Surgery

Before surgery, make sure you know when to stop eating and drinking and which medications to take and not to take on the day of surgery. In general, most people will be asked to stop eating and drinking the midnight before surgery. In general, you will be asked not to take most of your medications except beta blockers. Check with your bariatric surgery team for specific instructions.

On the day of surgery, arrive at the hospital about 2 hours before surgery. Bring your identification card and insurance card. You will go to a special area to prepare for surgery. It is normal to feel anxious or scared. Please ask the people taking care of you if you need help in any way.

You will be visited by nurses and doctors that may include:

- Your surgeon
- Your anesthesiologist, the doctor who will keep you safely asleep during surgery
- Your pre-surgery nurse, who will prepare you for surgery
- Your circulator nurse, who will be in the room with you during surgery

You may be asked to review and sign a consent form for surgery if you have not already done so. You may be asked for contact information if you would like anyone notified after your surgery. This is a good time to ask any remaining questions before surgery.

The anesthesiologist will review their plan for keeping you safely asleep during surgery. They will ask you to sign a separate consent form allowing them to take care of you. They may give you some medications to help you feel more relaxed before surgery.

The nurses will ask you questions about your medical history, medications, and the last time you ate or drank. This is all to make sure that it is safe for you to undergo surgery. They will ask you to change into a gown, check your vital signs, place a line into one of your veins, and may give you some medications. One of the common medications is an injection into the skin that helps to prevent blood clots.

Once it is time to go to the operating room, you will be taken there and asked to lay on the operating table. You will be covered with blankets to keep you warm. Since the bed is narrow, your arms and legs will be gently secured to the bed to keep you from falling. You will have special stockings placed on your lower legs that will squeeze them gently to prevent blood clots.

The anesthesiologist may give you medications to help you relax. He or she will use a mask on your face to gently give you extra oxygen. They will then give you more medications to help you go to sleep to not feel or remember anything during surgery. The surgery will begin after you are fully asleep. Everyone in the room has a duty to keep you safe and comfortable.

Next, we will discuss what to expect after your surgery is completed.

II.   What to Expect Right After Bariatric Surgery

After bariatric surgery is completed, you will be taken to a recovery unit. Here, nurses will monitor your pain level, how awake you are, your vital signs, and help to keep you warm and comfortable. If there are any problems, your doctors will be notified to be able to help you.

Once you are awake enough, you may be moved to a room in the hospital to keep recovering from surgery. You will have fluids going into your vein to keep you hydrated. You will have medications available to help to control pain, nausea, and to prevent blood clots. If you take any medications at home, some of these medications will be re-started and some may not. Ask your bariatric surgery team about your specific care.

What you may feel after surgery

You can expect to feel some nausea, bloating, and pain after bariatric surgery. Nausea and bloating usually go away within a few days. Pain usually improves day to day. Your pain level will not be zero. You will have pain medications to help control pain and will be encouraged to use medications that you can take by mouth.

Staying active right after surgery

You will be asked to stay active after surgery. Try to get out of and stay out as much as possible. You can walk and move around with help on the day of surgery. It may hurt to move, but it is very important to start moving soon after surgery.

Drinking liquids after surgery

You will start to drink liquids after surgery. The specific type and timing depend on your surgery and overall health. Ask your bariatric surgery team for your specific instructions. In general, you will start drinking liquids within a day of your surgery. The goal for most patients is to drink at least 64 ounces per day. This equals 8 cups of liquid per day.

You will not be able to drink a lot at once. The size of your stomach has changed. You will feel fuller faster. Drink small sips throughout the day. Drink at least 1 ounce every 15 minutes when you are awake. Keep track of this on a piece of paper or on your phone. There is an example of a paper tracker you can use in **Resources** at the end of this book.

Sometimes, you will feel very full. Do not push it. While you are in the hospital, you will stay on fluids by vein until you can drink enough liquids on your own. Remember that you will need to drink small sips throughout the day. Because your stomach is now smaller, you will not be able to catch up later if you drink too little early in the day.

Next, we will talk about the steps to get you home after your surgery.

III.   Your Pathway from Bariatric Surgery to Going Home

The path you follow between surgery and home is different based on your surgery and overall health. Check with your bariatric surgery team for your specific details.

In general, you will go through the next steps before going home:

- Be able to drink enough liquids to stay hydrated
- Have good enough pain control with medications you take by mouth
- Be able to urinate
- Be able to walk or move around at your baseline
- Have no signs of a surgical or other immediate medical problem
- Review your medications and instructions for home
- Prepare to go home

Only your bariatric surgery team can decide when you are ready to go home. Please be patient. We are trying to make sure that you are safe before going home.

Be able to drink enough liquids to stay hydrated

Being able to drink enough liquids to stay hydrated after bariatric surgery is essential. You will need to drink at least 64 ounces per day, equal to 8 cups of liquid. This helps avoid dehydration, which can make you very sick and need to return to the hospital.

Keep track of how much you drink. Aim for 1 ounce every 15 minutes while you are awake. You must be able to drink enough liquid on your own before it is safe to go home after bariatric surgery. If you are unable to drink enough liquids, you may need to stay longer in the hospital. There is an example of a way to track how much liquid you drink in **Resources** at the end of this book.

After your surgery, you will be on a schedule of liquid diets for a specific amount of time at home. Check with your bariatric surgery team for your specific instructions. We will discuss these different liquid diets in Chapter 4.

Have enough pain control with medications you take by mouth

It is reasonable to expect some pain from surgery. You will be offered different pain medications to use. Your bariatric surgery team may encourage you to try medications you can take by mouth because you can also take these medications at home.

Even with pain medications, your pain will not be zero. The goal of pain control is to be able to move around at your baseline, go about your daily life, and to be able to sleep. You must have pain under control on medications you take by mouth before going home after bariatric surgery.

Be able to urinate

It is very important to be able to urinate after bariatric surgery. Some patients can have difficulty urinating after surgery. When and how much you urinate may be tracked while you are in the hospital.

If you are having trouble urinating after surgery, there are a couple of things to try. Walking around and being upright can help. Medications can also help relax the right muscles to let you urinate.

If you are still unable to urinate, you may need to have a tube placed into your bladder that allows it to empty. This tube, called a Foley catheter, may need to stay in place when you go home. It can be taken out a few days later at the doctor's office to test if you can urinate on your own then. If you are going home with a Foley catheter, ask for instructions to make sure you understand how to take care of it at home.

Be able to walk or move around at your baseline

Moving around after bariatric surgery is essential. Movement helps with every aspect of healing, including pain control, avoiding blood clots, helping you to urinate, and keeping your muscles and joints active as you recover from surgery.

Get out of bed and stay out of bed as much as possible after surgery. This may mean means walking to the bathroom or around the unit often, staying upright in a chair, or using a wheelchair to get around if you used one before surgery. You can walk, go up and down stairs, do light exercise, and shower after surgery. You will need to be able to move around safely before going home after surgery.

These are some things to avoid for the first 4-6 weeks after bariatric surgery:

- Lifting anything over 20 pounds
- Strenuous physical activity that causes you to sweat or strain
- Soaking in water or swimming

Have no signs of a surgical or other immediate medical problem

Some patients do experience problems after bariatric surgery. These problems may include, but are not limited to:

- Bleeding
- Technical problems from surgery
- Not being able to drink enough liquids to stay hydrated
- Uncontrolled nausea or pain
- Blood clot
- Not being able to urinate
- Heart rhythm problems
- Kidney problems
- Other problems

While you are in the hospital, you may have your vital signs measured, samples of blood drawn and sent to the lab, and how much you urinate measured. These may all help to detect problems after surgery.

In a few cases, problems after surgery are treated by returning to the operating room for another surgery. Most problems after surgery can be monitored or treated with medications. If you have a problem after surgery, this may keep you in the hospital for a longer time. Your bariatric surgery team will work with you to help fix the problem and to get you home when you are safe.

Review your medications and instructions for home

Before you leave the hospital, you will review instructions to take care of yourself at home. You will review all new medications and any changes to your current medications.

You may have new medications after surgery to help control pain and keep your bowel movements regular. You may also have medication that lowers stomach acid production. The specific medications will vary by your surgery and your health conditions. Check with your bariatric surgery team about your specific medications.

There examples are listed as examples of common medications given to patients at home after bariatric surgery. Your bariatric surgery team may prescribe you a different set of medications:

- Pain medications
    1. Narcotic pain medications, such as Oxycodone
    2. Other pain medications, such as Tylenol®, Flexeril®, Gabapentin, and Lidocaine patches
- Stool softeners, such as Colace®
- Antacid medications, such as Protonix®

You may also be started on a medication to lower the risk of blood clots. These medications vary but may include Aspirin, Lovenox®, Xarelto® or others.

If you had any problems after surgery, you may be started on one or more new medications to treat these conditions. Make sure that you understand how to take these medications and the follow-up plan before you leave the hospital.

If you took any medications before bariatric surgery, these may have changed. Medication changes will be reviewed with you. Make sure that you understand how and when to take the medications that have changed. Medication changes are common for people with the following medical conditions:

- High blood pressure
- Diabetes
- Reflux
- Mental health conditions
- Breathing and lung problems
- Blood clots and heart problems
- Other health problems

Your discharge instructions will also explain how to take care of your incisions, your activity restrictions, your follow-up plan, and what to do if you have problems.

Your bariatric surgery team will give you their specific discharge instructions. For example, your bariatric surgery discharge instructions may include the following:

- Drink at least 64 ounces of fluids per day. Drink 1 ounce every 15 minutes while awake. Stay on your specific liquid diet schedule after your surgery.
- You can shower your incisions but do not soak them for 4-6 weeks after surgery.
- Do not lift more than 20 pounds for 4-6 weeks after surgery.
- You can walk, go up and down stairs, do light exercise, and have sex after surgery based on your comfort.

- Avoid strenuous activity that makes you sweat or strain in the 4-6 weeks after surgery.
- Review your medications before leaving the hospital and take them as prescribed.
- Follow up with your bariatric surgery team within 2 weeks.
- Follow up with your primary care doctor and specialist doctors within 1 month.
- If you are unable to drink at least 64 ounces of fluids per day, contact your bariatric surgery team.
- If you have worsening pain, nausea, breathing problems, a fever of over 100.4 degrees Fahrenheit, or have worsening redness or pain at your incision sites, if you are unable to urinate, or have worsening constipation or diarrhea, contact your bariatric surgery team.

Prepare to Go home

Before you go home, make sure that you understand:

- How to take care of yourself at home
- How to take your medications
- How much liquid to drink at home and what kinds to drink
- When you have follow-up appointments
- How to identify a problem at home and how to get help

You may be asked to call a family member or friend to come pick you up from the hospital. Before leaving the hospital, make sure that you know how to contact your bariatric surgery team if you have questions or problems at home.

In the next chapter, we will discuss life at home after bariatric surgery.

Chapter 4

Life After Bariatric Surgery

I.	**What to Eat After Bariatric Surgery**

What to eat right after surgery

After surgery, most bariatric surgery teams ask their patients to stay on a liquid diet for a specific amount of time. After bariatric surgery, the size of the stomach is changed. You will feel fuller faster and not be able to drink as much at once.

After bariatric surgery, it is important to start hydrated by drinking at least 64 ounces of liquid a day. Diet after surgery typically starts with liquids that are easy to swallow and require no chewing. You will slowly progress to thicker and more solid foods.

The exact diet and how long you stay on it after bariatric surgery may vary. Ask your bariatric surgery team for the specific details of your nutrition plan after surgery. Some will begin with clear liquids, while others may start with a different diet.

A common nutrition plan for the recovery period after bariatric surgery may be:

- For the first 2 weeks after surgery, start on a clear liquid diet
- For weeks 2–4 after surgery, advance to a full liquid diet
- For weeks 4-6 after surgery, advance to a soft diet

Let us review each of these liquid diets used after bariatric surgery:

- Clear liquid diet: any liquid that is see-through
- Full liquid diet: liquids, purees, and puddings that require no chewing
- Soft diet: liquids and soft foods that require very little chewing

Clear liquid diet (CLD)

Clear liquids are see-through and easy to swallow. If you hold the liquid up to a light and can see through it, it is a clear liquid. The clear liquid diet also includes some jelly products. It is a good idea to review the clear liquid diet with your nutritionist.

There is no breakfast, lunch, or dinner on the clear liquid diet. You drink these liquids all day, drinking at least 1 ounce every 15 minutes while you are awake. The goal is to drink at least 64 ounces per day after bariatric surgery. You can track your drinking on paper or online. There is a paper tracker example in **Resources** at the end of this book.

These are examples of foods on the clear liquid diet:

- Water
- Apple, cranberry, and grape juice
- Gatorade® and similar clear sports drinks
- Clear broth, including beef, chicken, fish, and vegetable broth
- Popsicles
- Clear protein drinks
- Jell-O® and similar clear gelatin products
- Tea and coffee in small amounts

Try to avoid carbonated drinks and caffeine after bariatric surgery. Carbonated drinks and caffeine may irritate your stomach, make you feel bloated, or make you dehydrated.

The full liquid diet is the next step up, allowing foods that have slightly more texture.

Full liquid diet (FLD)

The full liquid diet includes all liquids as well as purees and puddings that require no chewing. The full liquid diet is a step up from clear liquids by including thicker liquids and some semi-solid foods. If you have questions, it is a good idea to review the full liquid diet and any changes in your diet with your nutritionist.

These are examples of foods on the full liquid diet:

- All juice and water
- All smoothies with no chunks
- Pureed soup
- Pudding
- Yogurt
- Milk and cream
- Ice cream and custard
- Cream of wheat
- Protein drinks
- Pureed fruit and vegetables
- Baby food
- Food sauces with no chunks

At this stage, you will typically also start taking nutrient supplements. Work with your bariatric surgery team to find out exactly which supplements you need. Supplements typically include a multivitamin, calcium, B-complex vitamins, vitamin D, and iron.

The soft diet is the next step up, allowing foods that have mushy and ground texture.

Soft diet

The soft diet is also called the mushy diet or mechanical soft diet. On this diet, you can eat foods that are soft or mushy enough to not require much chewing. The soft diet includes all liquid and most mashed and ground foods. The soft diet is usually the last step before returning to food without any texture restrictions. If you have questions, it is a good idea to review the soft diet and any changes in your diet after bariatric surgery with your nutritionist.

These are examples of foods on the soft diet:

- Mashed potatoes
- Cottage cheese
- Cream cheese
- Oatmeal
- Eggs: scrambled, soft-boiled, and poached
- Ground meat and fish
- Gravy
- Mashed beans
- Avocado
- Bananas
- Hummus
- Tofu
- Peanut butter

As you advance to a soft diet, you will notice that not all things that you try are mashed, pureed, or ground very well. If something looks or feels too thick or too tough, do not eat it. Try to space out foods as you begin to eat them. You may notice that some foods work better than others. It may take time to adjust to which foods work best for you.

When you start eating a soft diet, it is easy to forget to drink enough liquids. Remember to drink at least 64 ounces of liquid every day.

Your nutritionist is the primary source of guidance for your diet before and after bariatric surgery. Please contact your nutritionist as part of the bariatric surgery team if you have any questions about your specific diet or face any problems in your nutrition.

What to eat in the long term after surgery

Bariatric surgery changes the size and shape of your stomach and changes how your body absorbs and metabolizes food. Learning how to deal with these changes is very important in keeping yourself healthy, hydrated, and full after bariatric surgery.

There are a few things to keep in mind about your nutrition after bariatric surgery:

- You will need to drink at least 64 ounces of liquid every day.
- You will not be able to eat or drink very much at once after surgery. Plan on smaller meals, more often throughout the day.
- You will need to take daily nutrient supplements.
- You may not like the same foods you did before surgery.
- Follow up regularly with your bariatric surgery team.

You will need to drink at least 64 ounces of liquid every day

After bariatric surgery, you will always need to keep yourself hydrated. This is not always easy to do with a busy schedule. In the beginning after your surgery, it is a good idea to keep track of how much you drink every day. There is an example of a paper tracker in **Resources** at the end of this book.

.

Start with 1 ounce every 15 minutes when you are awake for a goal of 64 ounces of liquid every day. As you adjust to the new size and shape of your stomach, you will discover how much you can comfortably eat or drink at any one time. When you start eating solid foods again, do not forget to keep drinking 64 ounces of liquid a day.

If you struggle with drinking enough liquids throughout the day or have pain or nausea when drinking, you need to contact your bariatric surgery team. This may be a sign of a problem that needs to be evaluated by your team.

You will not be able to eat or drink very much at once after surgery

Bariatric surgery changes the size and shape of your stomach. It also changes how you feel hunger, fullness and how your body absorbs and metabolizes food. As a result of all these changes, you will likely feel full faster than you did before bariatric surgery.

There is some planning involved in eating and drinking after bariatric surgery. Right after surgery, you will be on a liquid diet that progresses step-by-step, starting with foods that are easy to swallow and slowly adding foods that are thicker and more solid. During these steps, you will also start taking daily supplements, such as multivitamins, calcium, B-complex vitamins, vitamin D, and iron.

Once you are eating solid foods, it is a good idea to eat smaller meals more often throughout the day. There are no specific food restrictions in the long term after bariatric surgery. It is important to eat a variety of foods in moderation. Drink liquids often throughout the day, one sip at a time, for a goal of 64 ounces per day.

You will need to take nutrient supplements every day

After bariatric surgery, especially gastric bypass and duodenal switch surgeries, your body does not absorb nutrients as well as it did before surgery. For this reason, you will need to take nutrient supplements every day after surgery. The specific nutrients you need to take depend on your surgery and your overall health. Ask your bariatric surgery team about the specific nutrient supplements you need to take.

In general, you can expect to take supplements, such as a multivitamin, calcium, B-complex vitamins, vitamin D, and iron supplements after bariatric surgery. Most patients will be asked to undergo blood tests once a year to check their nutrient levels after bariatric surgery. This helps to identify any problems and keep your nutrition on track.

It is very important to take your nutrient supplements as prescribed because you can become very sick if you do not. For people who have not undergone bariatric surgery, taking supplements may be a choice. This is not so for patients who have had bariatric surgery. You will be required to take supplements for life. If you cannot eat or drink due to nausea, obstruction, or other medical problem, you may get dehydrated and low on some nutrients. If this happens, you need to contact your bariatric surgery team. You may need to be given fluids and nutrient replacement by vein in the hospital or clinic.

You may not be able to enjoy the same foods the same way before surgery

Bariatric surgery changes your physical body, how you feel fullness and hunger, your appetite, and how your metabolism and hormones work. These are complex changes. Many patients say that some taste differently to them after bariatric surgery. You may have liked carrots before surgery but dislike them afterwards. Once you are back to eating solid foods, you will discover which foods work best for you.

Follow-up regularly with your bariatric surgery team

Your bariatric surgery team will share your expected follow-up schedule. In many cases, you will follow up with your bariatric surgery team at least once in the first few weeks, then every few months, then once a year. The team will help you advance through the nutrition steps after surgery, supplements, and guide you in the long-term.

You have access to a nutritionist as part of your bariatric surgery team. It is a good idea to ask them for advice and support before and after your surgery. Many bariatric surgery teams also have patient groups and other resources with tips and advice from other patients who have had bariatric surgeries.

If you have medical conditions, such as high blood pressure, diabetes, high cholesterol, reflux, heart disease, arthritis, fatty liver disease, or kidney disease, it is important to continue to follow-up with a specialist doctor. You may have additional diet restrictions or nutrition requirements based on these medical conditions. It is best to ask your specialist doctor for details and to discuss your specifics with your nutritionist directly.

Next, we will talk about caring for your surgical incisions.

II.   How to Take Care of Your Incisions After Bariatric Surgery

Almost all bariatric surgery in the U.S. is done through small cuts through the front of the abdomen. Even when part of the stomach is removed, for example in a gastric sleeve, it is taken out through an incision that is typically one to two inches wide. The exact number and size of the incisions will depend on your surgery and overall health.

When you wake up from surgery, these incisions will be covered with waterproof surgical glue or with dressings.

If your incisions are covered with waterproof surgical glue, you can shower and gently wash the incisions with water and soap. Do not scrub the cuts. Keep the glue in place. The glue will peel off on its own in 1 to 2 weeks.

If your incisions are covered by dressings, these may not be fully waterproof. Before you leave the hospital, ask when the dressings will be removed and when you can shower.

Though you can shower after bariatric surgery without hurting your incisions, do not soak your cuts in water. Do not use pools, hot tubs, or swim for 4-6 weeks after surgery.

If you notice that any incision becomes red, warm to the touch, more painful, starts to drain, or has a bump that increases in size, contact your bariatric surgery team. You may need to have this incision evaluated for treatment. Ask your bariatric surgery team if you have questions about the care of your incisions.

Next, we will talk about staying active after bariatric surgery.

III.   How to Stay Active and Move Your Body After Bariatric Surgery

Staying active in the first 4-6 weeks after bariatric surgery

It is very important to start moving around soon after bariatric surgery. Movement helps you avoid blood clots, control pain, keep your muscles and joints active, and even helps to be able to urinate. Recovering from surgery happens faster by staying active.

I encourage patients to get out of bed and stay out of bed as much as possible after surgery. In the first 4-6 weeks after surgery, these are some good ways to be active:

- Walk around the house
- Go for short walks in the neighborhood
- Take the stairs, with support if you need it
- Eat and drink only when you are sitting or standing upright
- Use your wheelchair to move around often, if you used one before surgery

For the first 4-6 weeks after bariatric surgery, options for light exercise include walking, jogging, riding a bike, playing with kids or pets, and using light weights. When you exercise, remember to drink liquids to stay hydrated and to keep the exercise easy.

You can safely have sex after bariatric surgery. As with the rest of your activity, start slowly and carefully. If something does not feel good, stop and try something different another time. Avoid anything that makes you sweat or strain during the first 4-6 weeks after bariatric surgery.

For the first 4-6 weeks after bariatric surgery, here are some things to avoid:

- Lifting anything over 20 pounds
- Strenuous physical activity that makes you strain or sweat
- Swimming or anything that causes your incisions to become soaked
- Exercise that strains your abdominal muscles, such as crunches or planks

It is important to give your body time to heal during this recovery period of 4-6 weeks after surgery. As you adjust to the changes in your body, focus on staying hydrated, keeping track of your nutrition, and staying active with light activity every day.

Taking time off work after bariatric surgery

Most people take 1-3 weeks off work after bariatric surgery. How much time you take away from work depends on your surgery, overall health, recovery, and your work.

Discuss how much time you plan to take away from work with your bariatric surgery team. You may need lifting or other restrictions documented for your work. The team can provide you with the proper paperwork.

Staying active for life after bariatric surgery

About 4-6 weeks after your bariatric surgery, discuss your progress with your bariatric surgery team. If you have recovered well, they will determine when you can return to your regular activities. If you experience any problems after bariatric surgery, your recovery period may take longer.

After this recovery period, your activity is no longer restricted. It is a good idea to pace yourself after your recovery period.

If you start lifting weights, start low and slow. No matter what activities you choose, including walking, running, swimming, biking, abdominal muscle exercises, yoga, or anything else, start slow and be patient with yourself.

Focus on being active every day. Aim for any amount, for example 5-10 minutes at a time. It does not matter how fast or far you can walk or run or how many pushups you can do but rather that you do something sustainable and safe with your body every day.

When you exercise, it is important to stay hydrated. Do not forget to drink at least 64 ounces of liquid per day. When you exercise, drink more water to compensate.

Next, we will talk about when to call for help after bariatric surgery.

IV.   When to Call a Doctor for Help After Bariatric Surgery

People sometimes have problems after bariatric surgery. While you are recovering in the 4-6 weeks after bariatric surgery, call your bariatric surgery team for help if you are:

- Unable to keep liquid or food down
- Not able to drink 64 ounces of liquid per day
- Unable to control the pain in your chest or abdomen
- Feeling nausea that is severe or getting worse
- Having trouble breathing
- Have a fever of over 100.4 degrees Fahrenheit
- Having worsening redness, pain, or drainage at an incision site
- Unable to urinate
- Having constipation or diarrhea that is getting worse

Some of these problems can be addressed with a simple call to the office. Others may require a visit to the hospital. In some cases, additional surgery may be needed.

If your problem is not getting better and you are unable to reach your bariatric surgery team, you need to seek emergency care.

It is important to follow-up regularly with your bariatric surgery team and primary care doctor. No matter how long ago you had bariatric surgery, it is a good idea to contact your bariatric surgery team if you have the any of the following problems:

- Unable to eat or drink

- Strong pain in the chest or abdomen

- New or worsening reflux

- New or worsening nausea, vomiting or bloating

- Blood when you vomit or pass bowel movements

- Weight re-gain

These symptoms may signal a problem with your esophagus, stomach, intestines, gallbladder, metabolism, nutrition, or medications and should be evaluated by a doctor.

Next, we will talk about follow-up care after bariatric surgery.

V.   Your Follow-Up Care After Bariatric Surgery

You will have regular follow up with your bariatric surgery team after your surgery. In many cases, you will follow up with your bariatric surgery team at least once in the first few weeks, then every few months, then once a year.

The team will help guide you through the steps of your diet after surgery, nutrition supplements, monitor your progress, help you stay on track long term, and navigate any problems you may have.

You will continue to have access to a surgeon, nutritionist, nurses, coordinator, and in some cases, mental health and other specialists. Many bariatric surgery teams also have patient groups and other resources to help you stay on track and to get tips and advice from other people who have had bariatric surgery.

If you have medical conditions such as high blood pressure, diabetes, high cholesterol, reflux, heart disease, arthritis, fatty liver disease, kidney disease, or mental health conditions, it is important to follow-up regularly with a specialist doctor.

Next, we will talk about maintaining your health for life after bariatric surgery.

VI.   How to Maintain Your Health After Bariatric Surgery for Life

Now, we get to look at the big picture: How bariatric surgery may improve quality of life.

After bariatric surgery, your body may undergo changes in weight, appetite, metabolism, hormone activity, and medical conditions. Many patients take fewer medications, lower their blood pressure, and improve medical conditions including diabetes, cholesterol levels and heart disease. Many people can move around easier. All these changes may contribute to a better quality of life.

Keeping yourself healthy requires a lot of support. You have the support of a bariatric surgery team to help you reach your goals. Family, friends, and people who have undergone bariatric surgery can help provide help along your journey. Your primary care doctor, specialist doctors and mental health specialists are also powerful supporters in your health care for life.

Here are some guidelines for staying healthy in the long run after bariatric surgery:

- Drink at least 64 ounces of liquid every day.
- Eat a variety of foods throughout the day in smaller, more often meals.
- Take your daily nutrition supplements as prescribed.
- Stay physically active every day. Every action counts.
- Follow up regularly with your bariatric surgery team, primary care doctor, specialist doctors, and mental health specialist
- Contact your bariatric surgery team when you have a problem.

Chapter 5

Final Thoughts from a Bariatric Surgeon

I.   The Purpose of Bariatric Surgery Is to Improve Quality of Life

When we talk about health, we mean a lot of different things. Health includes genetics, medical history, health conditions, medications, weight, nutrition, physical activity, mental health, and our environment and policies. I think the most important consideration about health is qualify of life.

There are many reasons to consider bariatric surgery. Whether you are considering bariatric surgery to lose weight, change how many medications you take, to sleep better at night, to have less reflux, or to move around easier, all these reasons can make a difference in quality of life.

The number of pounds you weight matters much less than how your body works and makes you feel. The purpose of bariatric surgery is to help you feel better with a body that works better for you.

II.   Bariatric Surgery Is a Small Part of a Bigger Picture

Bariatric surgery is a small part of a much bigger picture. We all deserve access to good physical and mental health care. In bariatric health care, surgery plays a role, but so does overall health, medications, nutrition, physical activity, mental health, family, friends, community, and access to support along every step of the way.

For anyone considering bariatric surgery, I hope that this guide provides you with realistic support throughout the process. You are not alone, and no, you are not the only one with that question. Thank you for choosing this guide as one of the resources to support your journey to better quality of life.

There are additional resources listed in the following **Resources** section.

Resources

1. BMI calculator

2. Liquid tracker after bariatric surgery

3. Example of how to use liquid tracker

BMI calculator

Use this link to calculate your BMI using your height and weight:

https://www.nhlbi.nih.gov/health/educational/lose_wt/BMI/bmicalc.htm
Published by NIH.gov

You can also do the calculation on your own.

Take your weight in kilograms and divide it by your height in meters squared:
BMI = kg/ m^2

BMI categories:

BMI	Category	Qualifies for bariatric surgery
Less than 18.5	Underweight	No
18.5-24.9	Normal weight	No
25-29.9	Overweight	No
30-34.9	Obesity, level I	Usually no
35-39.9	Obesity, level II	Yes, if have some medical conditions
40 or over	Obesity, level III	Yes

Liquid tracker after bariatric surgery

Date				
	Ounce 1	Ounce 2	Ounce 3	Ounce 4
MIDNIGHT				
1:00 AM				
2:00 AM				
3:00 AM				
4:00 AM				
5:00 AM				
6:00 AM				
7:00 AM				
8:00 AM				
9:00 AM				
10:00 AM				
11:00 AM				
NOON				
1:00 PM				
2:00 PM				
3:00 PM				
4:00 PM				
5:00 PM				
6:00 PM				
7:00 PM				
8:00 PM				
9:00 PM				
10:00 PM				
11:00 PM				

Example of how to use the liquid tracker after bariatric surgery

Date	Monday, 6/6/2021			
	Ounce 1	Ounce 2	Ounce 3	Ounce 4
MIDNIGHT				
1:00 AM				
2:00 AM				
3:00 AM				
4:00 AM				
5:00 AM				
6:00 AM				
7:00 AM	X	X	X	X
8:00 AM	X	X	X	
9:00 AM	X	X	X	X
10:00 AM	X	X	X	X
11:00 AM		X	X	
NOON	X	X	X	X
1:00 PM	X	X	X	X
2:00 PM	X		X	X
3:00 PM	X	X	X	X
4:00 PM				
5:00 PM				
6:00 PM				
7:00 PM				
8:00 PM				
9:00 PM				
10:00 PM				
11:00 PM				

Citations

1. Arterburn DE, Telem DA, Kushner RF, Courcoulas AP. Benefits and Risks of Bariatric Surgery in Adults: A Review. JAMA. 2020 Sep 1;324(9):879-887. doi: 10.1001/jama.2020.12567. PMID: 32870301.

2. Bettini S, Belligoli A, Fabris R, Busetto L. Diet approach before and after bariatric surgery. Rev Endocr Metab Disord. 2020 Sep;21(3):297-306. doi: 10.1007/s11154-020-09571-8. Erratum in: Rev Endocr Metab Disord. 2020 Aug 17;: PMID: 32734395; PMCID: PMC7455579.

3. Behary P, Miras AD. Food preferences and underlying mechanisms after bariatric surgery. Proc Nutr Soc. 2015 Nov;74(4):419-25. doi: 10.1017/S0029665115002074. Epub 2015 May 20. PMID: 25990312.

4. Calculate your body mass index. NIH. Accessed August 2022. Website URL: https://www.nhlbi.nih.gov/health/educational/lose_wt/BMI/bmicalc.htm

5. Chang SH, Stoll CR, Song J, Varela JE, Eagon CJ, Colditz GA. The effectiveness and risks of bariatric surgery: an updated systematic review and meta-analysis, 2003-2012. JAMA Surg. 2014 Mar;149(3):275-87. doi: 10.1001/jamasurg.2013.3654. PMID: 24352617; PMCID: PMC3962512.

6. Collazo-Clavell ML, Clark MM, McAlpine DE, Jensen MD. Assessment and preparation of patients for bariatric surgery. Mayo Clin Proc. 2006 Oct;81(10 Suppl):S11-7. doi: 10.1016/s0025-6196(11)61176-2. PMID: 17036574.

7. Courcoulas AP, King WC, Belle SH, Berk P, Flum DR, Garcia L, Gourash W, Horlick M, Mitchell JE, Pomp A, Pories WJ, Purnell JQ, Singh A, Spaniolas K, Thirlby R, Wolfe BM, Yanovski SZ. Seven-Year Weight Trajectories and Health Outcomes in the Longitudinal Assessment of Bariatric Surgery (LABS) Study. JAMA Surg. 2018 May 1;153(5):427-434. doi: 10.1001/jamasurg.2017.5025. PMID: 29214306; PMCID: PMC6584318.

8. de Raaff CAL, Gorter-Stam MAW, de Vries N, Sinha AC, Jaap Bonjer H, Chung F, Coblijn UK, Dahan A, van den Helder RS, Hilgevoord AAJ, Hillman DR, Margarson MP, Mattar SG, Mulier JP, Ravesloot MJL, Reiber BMM, van Rijswijk AS, Singh PM, Steenhuis R, Tenhagen M, Vanderveken OM, Verbraecken J, White DP, van der Wielen N, van Wagensveld BA. Perioperative management of obstructive sleep

apnea in bariatric surgery: a consensus guideline. Surg Obes Relat Dis. 2017 Jul;13(7):1095-1109. doi: 10.1016/j.soard.2017.03.022. Epub 2017 Mar 30. PMID: 28666588.

9. Estimate of Bariatric Surgery Numbers, 2011-2020. ASMBS. Published June 2022. Accessed August 2022. Website URL: https://asmbs.org/resources/estimate-of-bariatric-surgery-numbers

10. Gebran SG, Knighton B, Ngaage LM, Rose JA, Grant MP, Liang F, Nam AJ, Kavic SM, Kligman MD, Rasko YM. Insurance Coverage Criteria for Bariatric Surgery: A Survey of Policies. Obes Surg. 2020 Feb;30(2):707-713. doi: 10.1007/s11695-019-04243-2. PMID: 31749107.

11. Gill H, Kang S, Lee Y, Rosenblat JD, Brietzke E, Zuckerman H, McIntyre RS. The long-term effect of bariatric surgery on depression and anxiety. J Affect Disord. 2019 Mar 1;246:886-894. doi: 10.1016/j.jad.2018.12.113. Epub 2018 Dec 28. PMID: 30795495.

12. Hachem A, Brennan L. Quality of Life Outcomes of Bariatric Surgery: A Systematic Review. Obes Surg. 2016 Feb;26(2):395-409. doi: 10.1007/s11695-015-1940-z. PMID: 26494369.

13. Katz JN, Selzer F, Robinson MK. Bariatric surgery and pain outcomes in osteoarthritis. Osteoarthritis Cartilage. 2021 Oct;29(10):1383-1385. doi: 10.1016/j.joca.2021.07.004. Epub 2021 Jul 30. PMID: 34339823.

14. Major P, Stefura T, Dziurowicz B, Radwan J, Wysocki M, Małczak P, Pędziwiatr M. Quality of Life 10 Years After Bariatric Surgery. Obes Surg. 2020 Oct;30(10):3675-3684. doi: 10.1007/s11695-020-04726-7. Epub 2020 Jun 13. PMID: 32535784; PMCID: PMC7467960.

15. Mechanick JI, Apovian C, Brethauer S, Garvey WT, Joffe AM, Kim J, Kushner RF, Lindquist R, Pessah-Pollack R, Seger J, Urman RD, Adams S, Cleek JB, Correa R, Figaro MK, Flanders K, Grams J, Hurley DL, Kothari S, Seger MV, Still CD. Clinical Practice Guidelines for the Perioperative Nutrition, Metabolic, and Nonsurgical Support of Patients Undergoing Bariatric Procedures – 2019 Update: Cosponsored by American Association of Clinical Endocrinologists/ American College of Endocrinology, The Obesity Society, American Society for Metabolic & Bariatric Surgery, Obesity Medicine Association, and American Society of

Anesthesiologists – Executive Summary. Endocr Pract. 2019 Dec;25(12):1346-1359. doi: 10.4158/GL-2019-0406. Epub 2019 Nov 4. PMID: 31682518.

16. Oates JR, Sharma S. Clear Liquid Diet. 2022 Jun 11. In: StatPearls [Internet]. Treasure Island (FL): StatPearls Publishing; 2022 Jan–. PMID: 30860735.

17. Range TL, Samra NS. Full Liquid Diet. 2022 Mar 9. In: StatPearls [Internet]. Treasure Island (FL): StatPearls Publishing; 2022 Jan–. PMID: 32119276.

18. Rubino F, Puhl RM, Cummings DE, Eckel RH, Ryan DH, Mechanick JI, Nadglowski J, Ramos Salas X, Schauer PR, Twenefour D, Apovian CM, Aronne LJ, Batterham RL, Berthoud HR, Boza C, Busetto L, Dicker D, De Groot M, Eisenberg D, Flint SW, Huang TT, Kaplan LM, Kirwan JP, Korner J, Kyle TK, Laferrère B, le Roux CW, McIver L, Mingrone G, Nece P, Reid TJ, Rogers AM, Rosenbaum M, Seeley RJ, Torres AJ, Dixon JB. Joint international consensus statement for ending stigma of obesity. Nat Med. 2020 Apr;26(4):485-497. doi: 10.1038/s41591-020-0803-x. Epub 2020 Mar 4. PMID: 32127716; PMCID: PMC7154011.

19. Samson R, Ayinapudi K, Le Jemtel TH, Oparil S. Obesity, Hypertension, and Bariatric Surgery. Curr Hypertens Rep. 2020 Jun 26;22(7):46. doi: 10.1007/s11906-020-01049-x. PMID: 32591918.